Your Heart
IS
Your Health!

by

Robert "Bob" Butler

ISBN #978-1-329-59258-2

Dedication

This "book" is dedication to my doctors, who listened when I spoke and found the source of my complaint. Without their diligence, I would most likely have dropped dead to the surprise of my family. I thank them and hope that my writing this may help to save others who have no idea that they are in danger.

Prologue

First, let me emphasize: I AM NOT A MEDICAL PROFESSIONAL! This is written by a layman who has been so inspired by his experience that he has chosen to try to inform, though without expertise or a medical background, to tell others the simple, basic facts that he has learned and which everyone should know about staying healthy and, especially, caring for the most important organ in the body, THE HEART! Without it, nothing else works! I am NOT an expert, but I hope that you will read this and take it to heart (pun intended)! I will not preach or beg or insult you. I only want you to think about your heart, what you put into your body to keep it healthy, and what you do to keep it strong. This book is as simple as that!

If you want expert material, you can find plenty of that on the internet, at your doctor's office, or at the public library. The American Heart Association is a great source of detailed information if you need that. I strongly suggest that you include a visit to the cardiologist to your annual check-up list!

I will try to write this with humor so that you won't get too bored and ignore the important message. Feel free to pass this book along or copy pages of it to give to friends so that they can benefit also. It is my intention that this booklet should be FREE to everyone. All that you have to do is read it, think about it, and act upon what you feel is important to you. I wish each of you a LONG and happy "heart life!"

My Story

Hi, I'm Bob. I was a runner for 30+ years, not competitively but for health, relaxation, and because I enjoyed it. I have never smoked in my life. I have eaten my share of cookies, ice cream, cake, hamburgers, French fries, etc., though I had given up most red meat the past ten years. I drank very little alcohol in my life. I probably averaged a couple of six packs a year (once I was of legal age, naturally!). I have never used illegal drugs or abused prescription drugs. I never had the urge or felt the need. The only thing in my life that I thought might be a problem for me was stress, which was part of the reason that I watched my weight and ran. I never have had a problem with my cholesterol levels. As a matter of fact, a few months before I began to feel a "flutter or twitch" in my chest (nothing painful just odd), my doctor had done the annual blood work and told me that my results were "unusually normal." We laughed at that.

About a month later, I went to my doctor (his nurse practitioner, actually) and complained about the "flutter," so she scheduled me to wear a "holter monitor" for 24 hours. When the doctor's office called me to tell me that I had an appointment with a cardiologist, my suspicions were vindicated that it was my heart and not indigestion. The cardiologist sent me for an echo cardiogram, which turned out to be perfectly normal. However, because my father had been through by-pass surgery, he suggested a cardiogram. That was fine with me. I did not like the "fluttering" feeling in my chest.

On May 18th, 2015, I went to the hospital and was told that I'd either wake up in the recovery room to go home or in I.C.U. because I probably had gotten a stent. It was a great experience for me. The cath lab people were so nice and professional, and I then went to sleep for the procedure, at least I think that's what happened. After you've been given "versed," (the drug which actually causes amnesia), even if you were awake it's no longer in your memory. I woke up in the I.C.U. and found out that I'd gotten two stents, prox and mid LAD, whatever that means. I wasn't exactly shocked, but I never thought that I'd have any blockages. I have always tried my best to take good care of my body. The cardiologist explained that because of genetics, I was prone to the type of plaque that had built up in my arteries. My lifestyle did help, probably kept me from dropping dead, but it was going to happen in my case.

Of course, I have since informed my son and daughters of the risks that the family genes pose for them in the future so that they will be aware and can watch for signs of heart disease more closely. I strongly suggest that you find out about your genetic makeup now so that you can make changes if necessary and be alert to the warning signs which might appear, such as my "heart flutters."

Just because your family history may not seem to pose you a great risk doesn't mean that you can just ignore plaque buildup in your arteries. Your eating and exercising habits can most definitely still put you at risk. It doesn't mean that you have to eat oatmeal every morning, a dry salad for lunch, and steamed, tasteless veggies with a small portion of oven baked fish or chicken every night to avoid cholesterol dangers. It just means that you should be more moderate in all aspects of your eating habits.

Food-the Non-drug Abuser's *Cocaine/Heroin*

Before I get into the "meat" of this book, I must add this observation. The foods that we consume can be healthful and helpful in providing us the energy that we need to live long and vibrant lives. However, many of the things which we put into our bodies are just as addictive and just as dangerous as any illegal drug on the street today, when taken in large amounts without an equal addition of exercise and relaxation. *Sugar, salt, caffeine, and fat are just as addictive as those dangerous drugs about which we are always warned.*

Sodium

Okay, first thing up for "bad" things to avoid is that tasty, wonderful **SALT**! You might say, "We need salt in our diet to retain fluid." Correct, but you don't need to add salt to your food to get what you need. The fact is most packaged foods contain 5 to 10 times the amount of salt that is needed, much less safe. Sodium is one of those ingredients that is listed on food packaging, thanks to the F.D.A.(I think). If there's much more than 100 mg per serving, watch out!

So, what's the harm in all that sodium/salt? It mostly raises your blood pressure, one of those silent killers that we hear about from the doctor. You cannot tell your own blood pressure by how you feel. A medical professional can't tell either by the way you tell him/her that you feel; that's why it's one of those standard things done when you visit the doctor and now some dentists. If your blood pressure is over 110/89, it is in the danger zone. The second number is the most important, but the other can be an issue too. One of the best ways to help keep down your blood pressure is to limit sodium intake to less than 1500 mg per day.

Yes, I know that salt puts the taste in your food, but there are ways to season foods without salt. There's a whole section in the grocery store devoted to seasonings. Look at them. I like to use rosemary, garlic, basil, and hot sauce to season my foods now, but I'm still experimenting. Search the internet for "seasoning without salt" recipes and suggestions. We all know that everything is on the internet now! For me, the answer has been **HOT SAUCE**, which does contain some sodium. Just be careful which brand of **HOT SAUCE** you buy. Spicy foods with low sodium are more enjoyable and healthier anyway!

Yes, I know sea salt is supposed to be the answer, but it's still salt with sodium. If you don't have blood pressure issues, it's better to start eliminating that extra sodium from your diet now than wait until you wake up one day stuffing one of the many blood pressure medicines down your throat.

I will have more to say about sodium in other sections, primarily foods eaten out of the home and snack foods, one of the great pleasures in life. Of course, great pleasures come with not-so-great side effects sometimes.

Fats

Another of the **Big Three (caffeine being separate issue)** which make up our tasty eating habits, not the healthiest most people will admit, is **fat.** Don't be confused by the various categories or fat: polyunsaturated, saturated, mono-saturated, and the worst of the bunch, **trans fats.** They are **all** fats, just some are healthier for you than others. Yes, the body does need fat, but not at the levels that most people consume. It's really scary if you look at foods. Again, thank the F.D.A. for requiring nutritional labels on packaged foods.

Why is fat bad for you? There are two main reasons. The first is weight gain, which puts an extra strain on your heart. Imagine walking around with a 25 pound weight hanging off your body all day long. That extra weight makes your heart have to work harder just to keep the body operating at normal limits. What if you're 50 pounds overweight? Imagine being 100 or more pounds overweight and what that would be like trying to just walk. The heart would be stressing, angry at you for making it work so hard.

The other reason is that fats, along with cholesterol, raise your LDL, low-density lipoprotein cholesterol levels. That can lead to the build up of plaque in your coronary arteries, and THOSE are the things which provide your muscles and heart with oxygenated blood! Given enough time, the plaque will harden and narrow the coronary arteries. What happens when you squeeze a garden hose? Less water comes out and what does is spewing, not flowing normally. That's what happens when you have high blood pressure, which can lead to a heart attack. It can lead to other problems as well, but you get the picture, right? **Eating an excessive amount of fatty foods is bad!**

How much is too much for you? Depends on many things, but keep in mind that I was a runner for 30 years. My heart rate is in the low 50's. Sounds good, but I had a blockage. I ate too much fatty foods, even the good kind. Talk to your doctor about what limits you should put on your fat intake.

Sugar

Ah, yes, the most wonderful part of our diet, sugar! Donuts, cookies, cakes, ice cream, pudding, pies, soft drinks, etc. What would life be without sugar? It is the **third of the diet devils**, along with salt and fat. Can you imagine cooking without these things. You don't have to eliminate them entirely, just moderate them.

We all know the worst part of eating all that sugar: **diabetes**, right? Well, there are other side effects, the greatest of which is weight gain (remember that angry heart!), which leads to all sorts of health issues, including heart disease and diabetes.

Most of the enemy is easily seen: cookies, pies, cakes, etc. but there are many others. Check the labels of most all foods, including breakfast cereals, a staple in the American breakfast. Sure, it's fast in the morning for kids, but there are healthy alternatives. One of the hardest addictions to break is sugar. The only two which are worse, maybe, are caffeine and smoking.

Nearly as I can figure, using the internet, maximum grams of sugar each day should be about 30. Men apparently can tolerate a little more than women. Best thing that I know to do is use *Stevia* in place of sugar or those nasty chemicals in the artificial sweeteners.

Caffeine?

I used to think that there were only three "bad" parts of our diet, but that was before my own experience, before I learned what caffeine does to the heart. Yes, that "jump start" which drinking coffee and tea and certain soft drinks give you IS a great feeling, especially in the morning; years of doing that can lead to heart problems. I grew up with a disdain for breakfast because it made my stomach "unhappy," which led to early day "bathroom distress," as I called it.

Instead of eating bacon and eggs or oatmeal or cereals, I'd grab a Mountain Dew or Dr Pepper or Pepsi (after living in South America during my early years and getting tired of nothing but Coca Cola, especially the extra-sweet formula that was used in those days there) and use that "jump start" of caffeine and sugar to carry me through till lunch. It worked for me for years. Of course, I was younger and energetic and burned a lot of calories, so I never realized what the long-term impact of all that caffeine was doing to my heart.

Consuming caffeine is like "jump starting a car battery!" It sends a jolt of power, much like adrenalin, to the heart. Well, if you do that over and over again, everyday, it takes a toll on your heart's "nervous system." With me, it led to PVC's and SVT's, those extra heartbeats, those jolts that drive the heart crazy. It's almost like the heart gets out of sync with itself. Eventually it can lead to arrhythmia and heart attack.

Again, I'm no doctor, but artificially sending chemical shocks to the heart can't be good. Doctors only use the "paddles" or "defibrillators" when absolutely necessary to shock the heart back into rhythm. If it were safe to do on a constant basis, we could buy one to take home for game night!

Caffeine in daily quantities over long periods of time is not healthy for the human heart. Do yourself and your heart a favor and at the very least cut down your consumption of coffee and tea and soft drinks, or at least use de-caffeinated versions of those drinks. Also, remember that chocolate has caffeine too, although less. White chocolate has none. Do a little research and find out what works best for you, but **please reduce or eliminate caffeine from your diet!**

Smoking

I can't believe that I even need to
mention this, but I will. Not having been
a smoker, I don't get it, the need to
smoke. I do understand the addictive
power of nicotine and whatever else is in
tobacco. If you aren't concerned about
what smoking does to your lungs, consider
what it does to your heart!

First, to no one's surprise, smoking
reduces the amount of oxygen that goes
into the lungs and thus the heart.
Second, smoking does to your heart what
caffeine does to your heart, speeds it up
faster than it should be for no good
reason. Third, smoking obviously (at least
to me) raises your blood pressure, and we
all know how wonderful high blood
pressure is! Fourth, and maybe the
worst, it increases the plaque buildup

inside your blood vessels, thus creating a situation where a blockage is much more likely. Everyone knows what happens when the blood vessels stop pumping blood! Finally, blood clots are much more likely among smokers; blood clots can lead to strokes and heart attacks and death.

I can't tell you how many times that I've seen smokers out walking and jogging, not to mention their high pressure hobbies and jobs. The two activities do not mix. Help is available, and they can work! If you don't smoke or have already stopped, *do not smoke again!* If you are smoking, do your heart a favor and *stop smoking now!*

Cholesterol

I just thought of a great mantra that everyone should use. *You can't run away from your DNA!* I'm a perfect example of how true that statement is. I inherited the tendency for coronary heart disease. I did lots of things right, but I did enough of them wrong to end up in the cath lab. Without getting into a scientific discussion explaining cholesterol and how it works, the key is to see a doctor regularly, have your blood work done regularly, and change your diet so that cholesterol is less of an issue for you. It really doesn't matter who you are or what your family history is, cholesterol screening should be done at least annually. My doctor tells me that there is a cholesterol test that can be done but insurance companies don't currently pay for it. It can break down your cholesterol into the *MANY* kinds. There are so many more types than the standard LDL and HDL types. I didn't know this. Apparently with this test a person could actually target his/her diet to fight whichever negative cholesterol type that he/she has. It seems to me that insurance companies would be saving money by offering this test early so that people could begin fighting the problem before insurance is required to pay for constant drugs. I now take Simvastatin. It costs my insurance company **$230** a month for my prescription. I will be taking it for the next year, at least. It just seems more cost efficient to pay for the **$400** lab test and maybe avoid the drug down the road. Of course, what do I know!

Exercise

No matter what your preferred form of exercise is, **DO IT AND DO IT RELIGIOUSLY!** The internet it filled with sources that will help an individual find workouts and calorie-burning charts. I endorse reasonable exercise programs for everyone based on individual body mass and health. For me, though, the single most important exercise has been **WALKING**, a form of exercise which I have never liked. I believe the word is **"irony."**

I must say something about treadmills. I never really liked them before I spent twelve weeks in a cardiac rehab lab. Now, however, I am a big fan of treadmills. One way to get in lots of time walking is to put a good treadmill in your living room, right next to that recliner. Put on your favorite shows, climb on that treadmill, and walk your way to better health. You won't be sitting there, snacking chips and dip, along with a soft drink for three hours. Instead, you'll be burning calories AND enjoying an evening of television, if that's your evening entertainment.

I love to *run*, but after I came out of the cath lab, my cardiologist asked me not to run again until he thought that it was appropriate for me. I promised; after all, the man had just saved my life! From the end of May, 2015 until I completed cardiac rehab (September 14, 2015), I only walked. When the soreness was gone from my groin, I began walking a couple of miles, and after a week of that, I moved on to 5 miles, gradually increasing the pace. I didn't like not running, but I knew that my heart needed time to recover from the trauma of being invaded during the angioplasty. Within six weeks, I was walking 10 miles a day, even stretching it to 15 miles regularly, though my feet were not happy with me. My diet was strict, so the fat layer that had been covering my torso slowly began to melt away. Apparently there was also fat layers in my legs, but they are gone too. I am amazed! It only encouraged me to continue walking and avoiding those foods that I really enjoyed, though they were deadly.

I finally was allowed to resume running (jogging at first and listening to my body, something that I've always been good at) on September 14, 2015). I began by alternating laps of walking and jogging (where I walk requires 3 laps for a mile), and as of today (September 22, 2015), I am getting over the initial soreness in my quads and behind my knees so that I can run (jog really) easily. I'm in no hurry to sign up for a marathon (a goal that I'd given up on as my body kept telling me something wasn't right), but it is once again in the back of my mind.

My plan is to begin swimming three days a week (starting in January) and walking/running four days a week. I'm also adding some small hand weights to build up my arm and shoulder muscles for playing golf.

I understand that everyone can't work out three hours a day, but if you start with an hour in the morning and an hour in the evening, along with a good diet, your heart will be healthier, and you'll be preparing your body for a long, healthy life!

One more note: too much exercise is just as bad as not enough! DO NOT OVERDO IT, ESPECIALLY WHEN YOU ARE STARTING A PROGRAM!!

Calories

I've always been a big believer in monitoring my caloric intake. I'm not a fanatic about it, but I do little calculations in my head whenever I buy food, whether it's at the grocery store or a restaurant or a convenience store. There's an old adage: *To lose weight, you have to burn more calories than you eat!* I live by that!

Yes, there is a difference in where the calories originate when you think in terms of healthy eating. Excessive *sugar calories* can lead to problems, primarily diabetes! Inappropriate or excessive *fat calories* can lead to clogged arteries and a trip to the cath lab or worse, bypass surgery!

I can't tell anyone exactly how many calories his/her body needs each day to maintain a specific body weight. That can be calculated using the many charts and tables that are available on the internet. I only know that my ideal body weight for my height is 155 pounds. I'm working toward that slowly. That's the only healthy way to achieve such a goal.

Remember that **what you eat is** as important as **how much you eat!**

Remember too, *To lose weight, you have to burn more calories than you eat!*

Fast Food

One of the most wonderful yet deadliest innovations ever conceived by modern civilization is the *"fast food restaurant."* Their convenience has been a boost to post-World War II, and especially the post-Korean War, United States economy and lifestyle. As women became more and more a part of the workforce and two-income households became the norm, these low-cost, quick-meal food factories changed the way Americans ate. It also has led us to the national health crisis that we face today, unfortunately. Obesity, diabetes, heart disease, and the many other challenges which our society and our families have faced for years and now face into the future have their roots in this industry.

Teens, beginning in the 1950's and certainly still today, consume way too much of the deadly four (sugar, fat, sodium, and caffeine) as they frequent (much too frequently) fast food establishments. It's cheap, convenient, and a social scene, one which blue-collar and white-collar alike substitute for home-cooked, and what used to be better-balanced meals. It's not the fast food restaurants' fault that they've done such a great job promoting themselves and meeting the demand of the consumer. It's the nature of the beast; the beast, of course, is our society, workplace, and the social network of today!

However, that doesn't excuse the food industry from the blame which it must shoulder in the health crisis of today. *It is possible to create tasty, nutritious, balanced menus at a reasonable price!* The industry is just too lazy to do it! Some are making an attempt, but consumers aren't being demanding enough!

If fast food is an integral part of your lifestyle, then at least be smart about where you eat and what you choose from the menu. Most of the chains now have nutritional charts for their menu items on the internet, along with in the restaurants themselves (though that is rather inconvenient, especially when you have a limited time to eat). Spend a little time studying their menus and pick out the things which meet your needs. Send emails and use comment cards to inform your favorite chains that you'd like to see less sodium and fat and "meat alternatives" that can be healthier for you. Insist that they have caffeine-free drinks, especially those without sugar. Tell them to ask their soft drink suppliers to invest in new drinks that use *STEVIA* as a sweetener. Only when enough people ask enough times will the restaurants and food manufacturers comply. It has to be in their best interests. I guarantee that if you stop eating hamburger meat, that choice will soon disappear from their menus and be replaced with something better!

Look at all types of foods. Every chain, from burgers to oriental to Mexican to sandwich shops, use too much sodium, sugar, fat, and caffeine on their menus. If we stop eating those items, they'll get the message eventually and develop new menus which are healthier and more in demand.

Restaurants

Everything that I wrote about fast food menus in the previous chapter applies to traditional restaurants where foods are prepared to order. The great thing about these is that they are more responsive to their customers' desires.

Trained chefs certainly know how to prepare foods with less fat, lower sodium, and with less sugar and cholesterol. At least I hope that they are!

Ask what kind of oils are used in the foods that you wish to order. Tell the waiter that you'd like to see a nutritional chart of each menu item so that you can discern which ones are healthier for you. Insist upon low sodium, low fat (especially low saturated fat) dishes.

If your favorite restaurant can't do what you need, politely inform them that you will have to find another place that will. Since you are paying for what you

want, don't accept anything less!
Restaurants must adapt to consumers; it's
not for us to adapt to them!

Soft Drinks, Coffee, Tea, Etc.

I grew up drinking Coca Cola and Dr. Pepper and Mountain Dew and Pepsi and so many other brands. I just wish that they'd developed safer recipes over the years, especially as they saw the health trends that were developing. *IT IS TIME FOR THEM TO CHANGE!*

I think that their sales would skyrocket if just two changes were made. First, get rid of sugar/high fructose corn syrup (highly addictive sweeteners) and use *STEVIA* instead. If there is a cost consideration, buy up the Stevia production system, thereby controlling the price. Without a calorie problem, Americans (and the world) would be able to drink more soft drinks without the issue of diabetes or obesity being a problem for their products. Second, get rid of the caffeine. While I know that's a lot to ask, keeping consumers healthier for longer is a much better marketing idea.

The same issue holds for makers of coffee and tea. Caffeine is only kept in these products because it is an addictive substance justified because addicts (all those tea and coffee drinkers have been duped into believing that it's the great taste of the product that keeps them coming back for more) don't know any better. Sure, some caffeine is okay, maybe even healthful for the average person. At some point in the future, governments will be legislating the removal of these addictive features anyway, so it would behoove the industrial leaders to get ahead of the curve on this one.

Chips and Snacks

Man, do I love chips and snack crackers and popcorn and those Little Debbie cakes! I now limit myself to small packs (single serving only) of Frito's corn chips or some of the other lower saturated fat chips once a week or so. Baked chips with lowered fat content and low sodium content are my preference now, if I eat anything outside of my home foods at all!

Between the sugar, fat, and sodium contained in all of these snack foods, is it any wonder that there is an obesity, diabetes, and heart disease *epidemic* in this country! It has been observed that when any other culture has absorbed our dietary lifestyle, the people soon have the same medical issues that Americans do.

There are other ways to snack, but I'm not here to make those decisions for other people. I only point out that there are **HEALTHIER CHOICES THAT TASTE JUST AS GOOD.** It doesn't mean that you have to snack on apples and oranges. Personally, I eat an inexpensive brand of "animal crackers" during the evening as part of my drive to restrain from eating the "danger" snacks. Low in fat and sodium and sugar, these "cookies" allow me to enjoy a little sweetness without going overboard.

I know people who eat popcorn as their alternative snack food. The problem with popcorn is that the microwave versions not only have too much salt (the buttered versions have the fat problem), but the oils that they cook in have been found to be harmful. If you must do popcorn, at least pop your own the old-fashioned way, using healthier oil, or use an air-popping system. Avoid salting the snack, but if you can't handle that, at least use sea salt and very little of that.

Desserts?

Except for once a week as a treat (and then don't go crazy-you know, eating a whole cake or a pint of ice cream), this habit should be reserved for family holidays. I still enjoy pecan and pumpkin pies on Thanksgiving or Christmas, not to mention birthday cakes on those special days. However, the daily consumption of cookies, ice cream, cake, pies, etc. must be eliminated from your routine. Between the fat and sugar and sodium, that's how most people end up with daily insulin injections when they reach their "golden years," if they make it that long before diabetes catches up to them.

There are recipes which can be adapted to *STEVIA*, as well as use less salt and fat, but they don't taste the same. We all know it. Hopefully, the great chefs and bakers of the world will be inspired to create healthy versions that taste wonderful! I'm still waiting. Until then, I've found it easy to walk past this part of the store and the frozen dessert section, too! It takes time to develop the self discipline to do that, but a trip to the ER or the cath lab makes that discipline easier to find; I promise you!

BMI Charts/Bathroom Scales

My best advice is to visit the internet once to calculate and decide upon what your best weight and fitness level is for your body (considering your height). That being done, there's no point in looking over and over again, is there?

Bathroom scales aren't really needed if you are visiting your doctor on a regular basis. The nurses always weigh you and take your blood pressure. You'll know if your weight is going up or down by the way that your clothes fit, how you look in the mirror or the shower, or by the way your friends comment on your appearance. That number on the scale can only tell you how close you are to that magic number from the previous paragraph.

Once you are in a regular fitness/diet (diet meaning the food that you eat, not some arbitrary weight loss program) routine, you'll *FEEL HOW HEALTHY YOU REALLY ARE* without that number on the scale.

Keep in mind one thing. As you get older, your skin will not be as elastic as it once way, so you may lose all the fat that you need to lose but still think that there's more because of the skin folds. That takes more time as the body adapts to the loss of "filling" that stretched out the skin when you were carrying all that fat. If you're at your target weight, just keep exercising and eating right. Hopefully, the skin will get the message and shrink back to where you think that it belongs. If not, maybe you can afford a good plastic surgeon who can either remove it or tighten it somehow. Personally, I don't care because I know that I have returned my body to a *HEALTHY STATE.* Isn't that the point of all this anyway?

What Is My Secret Diet?

The secret is that there is no secret. I have merely selected the foods that work for me and contain the levels of sugar, sodium, and fat that I think are healthy for me. With the exception of whatever caffeine there may be in the occasional chocolate that I might consume (the only chocolate right now is in the *Silk Chocolate Soy Milk* that I consume, which is about the same as in decaf coffee), I don't get any other caffeine, period!

The following are the foods which I am currently eating. I am working on other items to vary my diet, but I'm in no hurry. These work well for now. By the way, you'll notice that there is no meat in my current home-prepared meals. I plan to add fish (salmon or something safe) and some chicken in the future.

Oatmeal (about half a cup dry) cooked in a microwave for 2 minutes and then

Milled Flaxseed added (heaping tablespoon). I add a few ounces of Silk Chocolate Soy Milk and one packet of Stevia for flavor. This was my daily breakfast an hour before I walk/run. Sometimes I don't consume anything before going out for my daily exercise.

After I return from exercise, I am now mixing one packet of Carnation Instant Breakfast powder (chocolate) into about 14 ounces of Silk Chocolate Soy Milk. I mix it in the blender so that it's like drinking a milkshake. This drink is high in protein, other vitamins, and calcium (more than regular milk). *HOWEVER,* **soy milk is not recommended for women (at least not much) to the extent that I use it because there is an indication that there is apparently an increased risk for breast cancer. Men should be aware that soy milk seems to show an increased risk of colon cancer.** I love what chocolate soy milk does for my weight control and fitness because of the levels of protein and calcium, so I will continue to use it. I use it and then don't for a time. I get bored eating and drinking the same things just like anyone would.

I cook a cup of brown rice seasoned with cayenne pepper and hot sauce as I need it for use with various vegetables and either black-eyed peas or field peas. A good gumbo recipe would be wonderful with brown rice. Just be careful of the sodium and fat content when seasoning the gumbo. This is also high in protein.

My spaghetti consists of combing a can of no-salt-added diced tomatoes (14.5 ounce can) in my blender with a regular-sized can of Hunt's spaghetti sauce while adding extra garlic and Italian seasonings, as well as hot sauce. It gets blended and then heated in a sauce pan. At the same time, I bring a pot of water to boil and add a 13.25 ounce package of WILD OATS brand Organic whole wheat spaghetti noodles and cook them for 7 minutes per package instructions. The noodles always come out exactly right. Once done, I drain the water and add the heated spaghetti sauce. This is enough for from 3-4 meals for me. While I'm not happy with the sodium content of the canned spaghetti sauce, by mixing it with the nearly-salt-free tomatoes, I dilute the sauce. Until I come up with my own reduced-salt recipe for spaghetti sauce that works for me, I live with a little extra sodium in this meal. Since I get so little sodium in everything else, I don't consider it a problem.

I find that a good alternative to brown rice is eating reconstituted mashed potatoes, leaving out the salt when bringing the water to a boil before adding the flakes. I use hot sauce and cayenne pepper instead of salt. If you have a flavorful seasoning combination (I prefer Tony's salt-free seasoning), use that in the water. I sometimes just eat the potatoes without adding veggies, squirting ketchup on the potatoes instead. My ketchup of choice is Hunt's without high fructose corn syrup.

The most important thing that I do everyday now is eat a cucumber or two with Greek salad dressing that I make. *I use apple cider vinegar, water, and olive oil combined with the Good Seasons Greek salad dressing packet spices.* It takes great, gives me the good oil that helps reduce the LDL cholesterol from my body, and provides the awesome benefits of apple cider vinegar (check them out on the internet).

I have experimented with a couple of vegan meatloaf recipes off the internet, and have found one which works fairly well. It consists of 50% black beans and 50% veggies (broccoli, squash, most anything colorful). Each are blended well in a food processor separately before being combined in a large bowl. I use raw oatmeal to bind it all together, mix in diced/ground up tomatoes (using a blender) along with lots of hot sauce and spices, including *lots* of garlic and olive oil. Once it is mixed and has some body, I spray a baking pan (any size or shape works) with cooking spray, pack most of in the pan and cook it at 375 degrees for 45 minutes. Any extra "meatloaf" that doesn't fit into the pan is pressed onto aluminum foil for "hamburger patties" and frozen for later. Actually, once the meatloaf is cooked, I let it cool, cut into pieces, and some is also put into the freezer for later. My meatloaf then becomes the protein for any meal, along with veggies, usually broccoli florets, my favorite side dish now.

The only time that I eat bread now is as part of a Subway sandwich (Although I do admire the alternative that Subway has provided people, the sandwich that you design is still only as good as your choices. Some of the ones advertised on TV are chocked full of sodium, fat, and cholesterol. I only eat veggies on whole wheat, *period.*) or a chicken salad sandwich that I get at Wally World if I just have to have something to eat when away from home. As far as other fast food restaurants, there are places which I visit (though rarely now), but I stick to grilled chicken sandwiches, *no fries or soft drinks*, and either bring my own drink or compromise with a diet-caffeine-free soft drink. My preference is *Diet 7UP*, which few carry.

For the past months, this is all that I eat. Perhaps that's the secret to my weight loss, along with all the walking! I have gone from about 185 pounds to 160 pounds so far.

Epilogue

Fast weight loss diets and extreme exercise programs can work, but the body, specifically the heart, can pay a heavy price for achieving goals using those methods. No one gets fat or out of good physical condition overnight. It takes years to go from a lean and active ideal body weight and fitness level to one that is almost the opposite, so you won't reverse things overnight either!

I don't recommend anyone do exactly what I have done. My method works for me. However, I do believe that with some discipline and good choices, anyone can achieve the goal of good health and reasonable fitness. I thought that I had been doing that my entire life, but it took the shock of learning that I had a blocked artery which required two stents to give me the incentive to go the extra step and take control of both my eating and exercising habits.

I'm not any smarter than anyone reading this book. I know that there may be health issues in my future that stem from old habits from my past. I accept that, but I don't accept that I won't be a healthier person by changing my exercise patterns and eating choices now. I've done that, and I promised myself that I wouldn't go back to the old ways. They obviously weren't enough to prevent heart disease. I might drop dead tomorrow, but it won't be because I didn't make good changes.

I hope that everyone who reads this book will do the same and make changes that work for him or her. It's really not that hard. A person just has to **want to change**!

About Me

I am currently retired and living in a small town in NE Arkansas named Marmaduke (funny thing is the school's mascot is Greyhound, not a Great Dane). I have a degree in business from what used to be called the University of Southwest Louisiana (Ragin Cajun's) but is now known as the University of Louisiana at Lafayette. I graduated from high school in New Iberia, Louisiana in 1969.

I am the divorced father of three and grandfather of four (at last count). I worked over the years as an accountant, a food service manager, a high school English teacher, and a night security officer, along with numerous other stints in various jobs. I spent a year as an AmeriCorps V.I.S.T.A. member in Cedar Rapids, Iowa, the year after the 2008 flood.

I have always wanted to be a writer, a publisher author actually. I have written a number of novels, screenplays, a stage play, a collection of short stories, and other things. I am self-published through LULU.com, but there are many other authors by the same name, so finding mine would be difficult without the following link.

http://www.lulu.com/spotlight/robertbutler

Shepherd's Inn: The Heart of Christmas

After the Snow Began to Fall

The Journey Home

Christin

From a Grandfather's Heart

The Courier: A Romantic Comedy

The Support Group

Essay Writing Made Easier

Short Stories by GEORGE

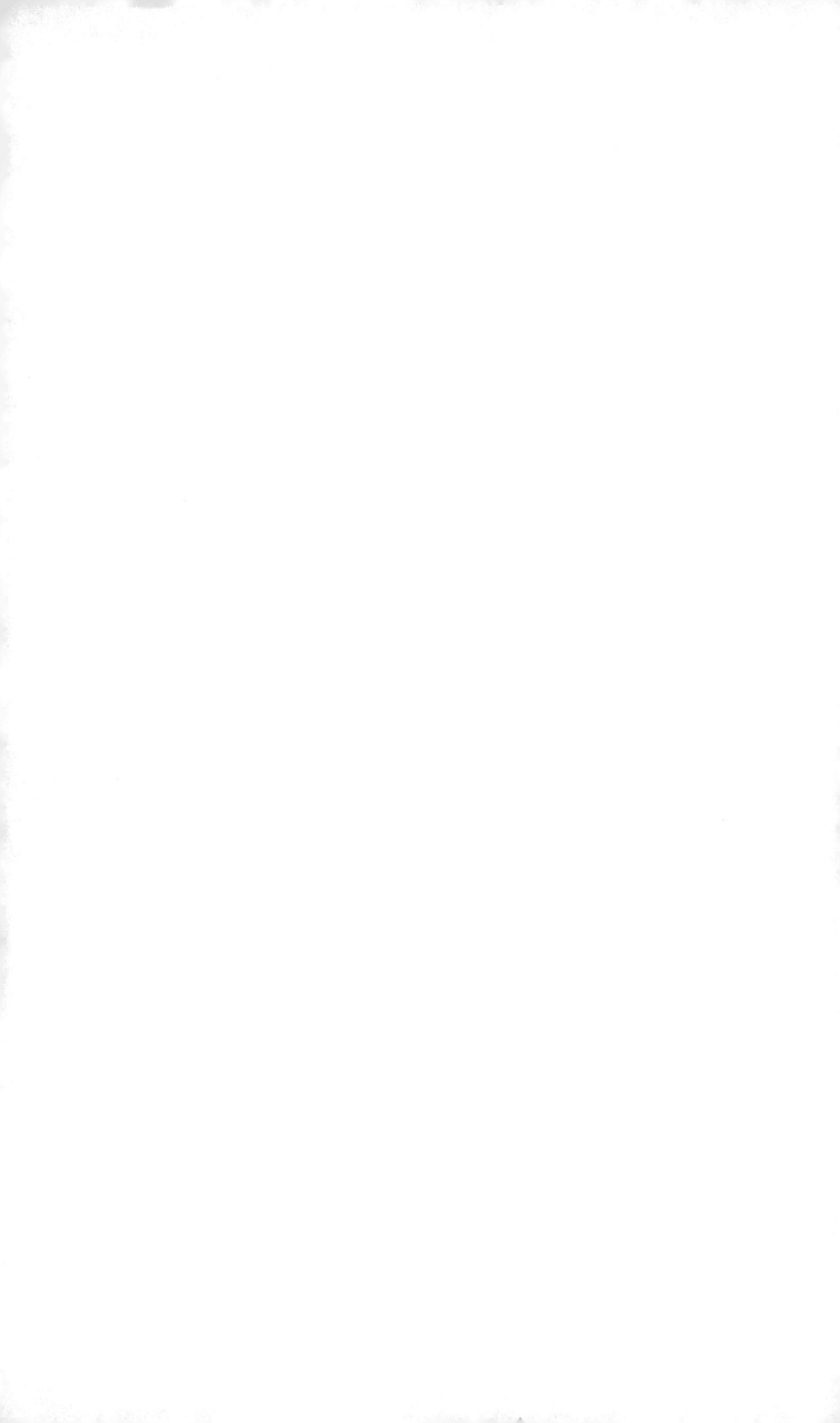